This book was compiled by Daniel Melehi
with the A.I assistance of Inventabot

<u>Dedication</u>
I hope this helps all of my wonderful
readers achieve all their goals in their
business. And I would like to thank my
wonderful wife for all of her continued
support in all my ventures.

©Daniel Melehi

May 7 2023

Contents

Chapter 2: Understanding Psychedelics.

Breaking the Stigma: Stories of Healing and Recovery with Psychedelics

Psychedelics have been a controversial topic for decades, but as scientific research continues to show promising results for their potential therapeutic benefits, it's time to break the stigma surrounding these substances. The purpose of this book is to share personal stories of individuals who have used psychedelics to aid in their healing and recovery process, as well as educate readers on the history, effects, and safety of these substances.

SUBCHAPTER 1.1: THE NEED TO BREAK THE STIGMA

For too long, psychedelics have been associated with counterculture and recreational drug use. This stigma has prevented individuals from seeking out potentially life-changing experiences and therapy. It's time to view psychedelics through a new lens, one that focuses on their therapeutic potential and the possibility of aiding those struggling with mental health issues. By breaking the stigma around psychedelics, we can open up a new avenue for individuals to seek help and treatment for their mental health struggles.

SUBCHAPTER 1.2: HISTORY OF PSYCHEDELICS

Psychedelics have been used for centuries in traditional healing practices and spiritual ceremonies. In the 1950s and 60s, they became popular in Western countries as a tool for personal and spiritual growth. However, as their use became more widespread, they also became associated with negative side effects and recreational drug use. This led to their criminalization in the 1970s, effectively ending most research on their therapeutic potential. Only in recent years have studies resumed, bringing renewed attention to the historical and cultural use of these substances.

SUBCHAPTER 1.3: LEGALIZATION AND RESEARCH

While psychedelics are still classified as illegal drugs in most countries, there has been some progress towards legalization and regulation for medicinal purposes. In the United States, for example, the FDA has granted breakthrough therapy designation to psilocybin for the treatment of depression. Additionally, research is ongoing in the fields of addiction treatment, PTSD therapy, and end-of-life care. These advancements offer hope for a future where psychedelics can be used as a legitimate tool in mental health treatment. Overall, Breaking the Stigma: Stories of Healing and Recovery with Psychedelics aims to educate the reader on a topic that has long been surrounded by controversy and misunderstanding. By sharing personal experiences and scientific research, we hope to contribute to a new understanding of the therapeutic potential of psychedelics and promote further study and exploration of their uses.

SUBCHAPTER 1.1: THE NEED TO BREAK THE STIGMA

In recent years, psychedelic-assisted therapy has emerged as a promising treatment option for a wide range of mental health conditions. Despite the promising research and positive outcomes reported by patients, there is still a significant stigma surrounding the use of psychedelics in a therapeutic context. This stigma is fueled by a lack of understanding and misinformation about psychedelic drugs. Many people still associate them with the counterculture movement of the 1960s and view them as dangerous and unpredictable substances. However, research has shown that, when used in a controlled setting with a trained therapist, psychedelics can be a safe and effective treatment for a number of mental health conditions. Breaking the stigma surrounding psychedelic-assisted therapy is essential if we want to explore the full potential of these drugs in a therapeutic context. Patients who are struggling with mental health issues need to feel safe and supported when seeking treatment, and the current stigma around psychedelics can discourage them from seeking help. Furthermore, the stigma can also impact the ability of researchers to conduct studies on the therapeutic potential of psychedelics. Many scientists struggle to get funding for their research due to the taboo surrounding these drugs, which can slow down the development of new therapies and limit our understanding of how these drugs work in the brain. Overall, it is crucial that we work to break the stigma surrounding psychedelic-assisted therapy. By doing so, we can help more people access safe and effective treatments for mental health conditions and unlock the full potential of these powerful drugs.

HISTORY OF PSYCHEDELICS

Psychedelics have a long history of use by various cultures for spiritual, medicinal, and recreational purposes. The earliest evidence of psychedelic use dates back to prehistoric times, with cave paintings in Africa depicting the ingestion of psychoactive plants. In South America, indigenous tribes have used ayahuasca for thousands of years in spiritual ceremonies, while North American indigenous cultures have used peyote for similar purposes. Psychedelics were also used in ancient Greece and Rome for religious rituals. The modern Western world's interest in psychedelics began in the

1950s and 1960s, when substances such as LSD, psilocybin, and mescaline became widely available and popularized by counterculture movements. Researchers at that time were studying the potential benefits of psychedelics in psychiatry and psychotherapy. However, due to their association with the counterculture movement and negative media portrayals, psychedelics were made illegal in the United States in 1970 with the passage of the Controlled Substances Act. This legislation hindered research on these substances for several decades. In recent years, the tide is turning as psychedelic research is regaining interest and support from the medical and scientific communities. The potential benefits of psychedelics for treating various mental health conditions including depression, anxiety, PTSD, and addiction are being studied in clinical trials. Many researchers believe that psychedelic-assisted therapy could represent a major breakthrough in the field of mental health treatment, offering a new and potentially powerful tool for promoting healing and recovery.

SUBCHAPTER 1.3: LEGALIZATION AND RESEARCH

The 20th century saw the prohibition of psychedelics, thanks to their association with the counterculture movement. However, recent years have seen a shift in global attitudes towards these substances. Countries like the United States, Canada, the Netherlands, Spain, and Portugal have made significant headway in decriminalizing and even legalizing psychedelics. In the US, cities like Denver, Colorado, and Oakland, California, have decriminalized or legalized certain psychedelic substances. In 2021, Oregon became the first state in the US to legalize the use of psilocybin, the active ingredient found in magic mushrooms, for therapeutic purposes. This shift towards legalization is in response to the growing body of research showing the therapeutic benefits of psychedelics in treating conditions like depression, anxiety, addiction, and PTSD. Researchers have found that these substances can promote neuroplasticity, allowing individuals to break out of harmful patterns of thought and behavior. Studies have shown that psychedelic-assisted therapy is particularly effective when combined with talk therapy and other forms of support. In fact, early research from the 1950s and 60s showed promising results in using psychedelics to treat alcoholism and other forms of addiction. Despite this, research was largely banned in the US and other countries in the 1970s. Today, there is a renewed interest in studying the potential of psychedelics in treating mental health conditions. Major universities like Johns Hopkins, NYU, and Imperial College London are conducting research on the therapeutic benefits of psychedelics. In addition, some companies like Compass Pathways and Mind Medicine are developing drugs based on psychedelics for use in treating mental health conditions. As more research is conducted and more countries move towards legalization, the stigma surrounding psychedelics is slowly being broken down. It is important to continue this conversation and explore the potential of these substances in promoting healing and recovery. This newfound interest in psychedelics has also led to a renewed conversation around ethics and safe use. As psychedelics become more mainstream, it is crucial that we prioritize safety and responsible use. This includes proper education, qualified guides or therapists, and support systems in place for individuals seeking psychedelic-assisted therapy. In the next chapter, we will explore the different types of psychedelics and their effects on the brain.

Chapter 2: Understanding Psychedelics

Psychedelics are a class of drugs that alter perception, mood, and cognitive processes.

This chapter aims to provide a basic understanding of the different types of psychedelics, their effects on the brain, and guidelines for safe usage.

SUBCHAPTER 2.1: TYPES OF PSYCHEDELICS

There are several different types of psychedelics, each with unique effects on the body and mind. The most well-known types of psychedelics include:

LSD (Lysergic Acid Diethylamide)

LSD is a synthetic drug that is known for its hallucinogenic effects. It alters the way the brain processes sensory information, leading to vivid and intense hallucinations. LSD is typically consumed orally in the form of tablets, capsules, or liquid drops.

Psilocybin (Magic Mushrooms)

Psilocybin is a naturally occurring psychedelic compound found in certain species of mushrooms. It has similar effects on the brain as LSD, but the intensity and duration of the effects are typically milder. Psilocybin is typically consumed by eating the dried or fresh mushrooms.

DMT (Dimethyltryptamine)

DMT is a naturally occurring psychedelic compound found in several different plant species. It is known for its intense and fleeting effects, which typically last less than an hour. DMT can be consumed through smoking or inhaling vaporized forms of the substance.

SUBCHAPTER 2.2: EFFECTS ON THE BRAIN

Psychedelics interact with the brain in several ways, primarily by binding to receptors for the neurotransmitter serotonin.

This leads to changes in mood, perception, and cognitive processing. The effects of psychedelics can vary depending on the substance and dosage, but they generally lead to altered sensory experiences, heightened emotions, and an altered sense of time and space.

SUBCHAPTER 2.3: DOSAGE AND SAFETY

Dosage is an important consideration when using psychedelics. The effects of psychedelics can vary greatly depending on the dose. It's essential to start with a low dose and gradually increase it over time to avoid overwhelming experiences. It's also important to use psychedelics in a safe and controlled setting, with people you trust and who are experienced with the substances. Psychedelics can be powerful allies in personal growth and healing, but they should always be treated with respect and caution.

TYPES OF PSYCHEDELICS

There are several types of psychedelics, each with its own unique chemical structure and effects on the brain. The following are some of the most commonly used psychedelics:

LSD (Lysergic Acid Diethylamide)

LSD is a powerful synthetic hallucinogen that was first synthesized in 1938 by Swiss chemist Albert Hofmann. It is typically taken orally and can produce intense visual hallucinations, vivid colors, and alterations in mood, thought, and perception.

Psiilocybin

Psiilocybin is a natural psychedelic compound found in certain species of mushrooms. It has been used for centuries in traditional religious ceremonies and can produce profound changes in perception, mood, and thought. It is typically taken orally and can produce effects that last for several hours.

DMT (Dimethyltryptamine)

DMT is a natural psychedelic compound found in certain plants and animals. It can be smoked, injected, or taken orally and produces intense visual and auditory hallucinations, euphoria, and changes in perception. The effects of DMT are typically short-lived, lasting only a few minutes.

Mescaline

Mescaline is a naturally occurring psychedelic compound found in certain cactus plants. It has been used for centuries in traditional religious ceremonies and can produce altered states of consciousness, euphoria, and changes in mood and perception. It is typically taken orally and can produce effects that last for several hours.

Ketamine

Ketamine is a dissociative anesthetic that can produce hallucinations and altered states of consciousness at high doses. It is typically used in medical settings for anesthesia and pain relief, but is also used recreationally for its psychedelic effects. Understanding the different types of psychedelics and their effects on the mind and body is important for anyone considering using these substances. It is important to note that the use of psychedelics can have real risks and potential negative consequences, and should only be done in a safe and controlled environment with proper guidance and support.

SUBCHAPTER 2.2: EFFECTS ON THE BRAIN

Psychedelics are known for their profound effects on the human brain. They work by altering the activity of certain neurotransmitters and receptors, which leads to changes in perception, mood, and cognition. Some of the most significant effects of psychedelics on the brain include:

Increased Brain Connectivity

Research has shown that psychedelic substances can increase the connectivity between different regions of the brain. This enhanced connectivity may explain the profound alterations in perception and consciousness experienced by users.

Increase in Neural Plasticity

Psychedelics also appear to increase neural plasticity, which is the brain's ability to reorganize itself in response to new experiences. This increased plasticity may be one reason why psychedelics have been shown to be effective at treating conditions like depression and addiction.

Activation of the Default Mode Network

The default mode network is a collection of brain regions that is active when the brain is at rest and not engaged in specific tasks. Research has shown that psychedelics can alter the activity of this network, leading to changes in self-referential thoughts and perceptions.

Increase in Serotonin Levels

Psychedelics work by interacting with serotonin receptors in the brain. Research has shown that the use of these substances leads to an increase in serotonin levels, which can have positive effects on mood, anxiety, and stress. In summary, the effects of psychedelics on the brain are complex and multifaceted. These substances can alter brain activity in profound ways, leading to changes in perception, mood, and cognition. However, more research is needed to fully understand the long-term effects of these substances on the brain and the potential risks associated with their use.

SUBCHAPTER 2.3: DOSAGE AND SAFETY

One of the most crucial aspects of using psychedelics for therapeutic purposes is understanding proper dosage and ensuring safety. Unlike with traditional medication, there is no one-size-fits-all approach to dosing with psychedelics. A variety of factors, including body weight, medical history, and current mental state, must be taken into account when determining an appropriate dosage. When using psychedelics in a therapeutic setting, it is common for a medical professional or licensed therapist to handle dosage and monitor the patient's experience. This ensures not only the safety of the patient, but also the effectiveness of the treatment. The professional can adjust the dosage as necessary based on the patient's responses, as well as provide emotional support throughout the experience. It is important to note that individual experiences with psychedelics can vary greatly. What may be a safe and effective dose for one person may not be appropriate for another. It is crucial to always start with a low dose and gradually increase as necessary, always with the guidance of a professional. In addition to proper dosing, safety measures must be taken to minimize the potential risks of using psychedelics. This includes ensuring that the environment in which one uses psychedelics is safe and comfortable, with minimal distractions or potential triggers. Additionally, it is important to have a trusted support system in place before, during, and after the experience. Overall, proper dosage and safety precautions are essential when using psychedelics for therapeutic purposes. Seeking professional guidance and support throughout the process can help ensure a safe and effective experience.

Chapter 3: Personal Stories of Healing

Psychedelics have gained increased attention in recent years for their potential to help individuals struggling with addiction, mental illness, and spiritual disconnection. In this chapter, we will explore personal stories from individuals who have used psychedelics as a tool for healing and recovery. Each story offers a unique perspective on the transformative power of psychedelics.

SUBCHAPTER 3.1: OVERCOMING ADDICTION

Addiction is a chronic and often debilitating disease that affects millions of people worldwide. While traditional treatment methods, such as therapy and medication, can be effective, they may not work for everyone. In this section, we will share stories from individuals who have used psychedelics as a means of overcoming addiction.

Breaking the Cycle

For years, John struggled with alcohol addiction, and traditional treatment methods failed to help him break the cycle. He turned to psychedelics as a last resort and was amazed at the transformative experience he had. He describes his trip as a wake-up call, where he finally saw the negative impact his addiction was having on his life and those around him. Since his experience, John has been sober for two years and credits psychedelics for helping him break free from the cycle of addiction.

Reconnecting with Purpose

Alicia had been struggling with opioid addiction for several years, and traditional treatment methods only provided temporary relief. She found herself stuck in a cycle of addiction, but after a psychedelic experience, she experienced a reconnection with her sense of purpose. She credits the experience with helping her realize the underlying issues driving her addiction and with giving her a new outlook on life. Today, Alicia is no longer using opioids and has found a renewed sense of purpose and passion for life.

SUBCHAPTER 3.2: COPING WITH MENTAL ILLNESS

Mental illness can be a debilitating condition that affects every aspect of a person's life. Traditional treatments such as medication and psychotherapy may not work for everyone. In this section, we will share personal stories from individuals who have used psychedelics to cope with mental illness.

From Darkness to Light

Ben had been struggling with depression for years and had tried everything from therapy to medication, but nothing seemed to work. He turned to psychedelics as a last resort and was amazed at the experience. During his trip, he experienced a sense of clarity and inner peace he had never felt before. Since his experience, Ben has been able to successfully manage his depression and live a fulfilling life.

Overcoming Trauma

Jenna had been struggling with PTSD for years and found traditional treatment methods to be ineffective. She decided to try psychedelics, which helped her to confront and process her traumatic experiences. She was able to move beyond the fear and pain and finally found the inner peace she had been searching for. Today, Jenna is no longer controlled by her trauma and has a renewed outlook on life.

SUBCHAPTER 3.3: FINDING SPIRITUAL CONNECTION

Many individuals turn to psychedelics not just for healing but to explore their spiritual nature. In this section, we will share personal stories from individuals who have used psychedelics to find a spiritual connection.

Connecting with the Universe

As a scientist, Ian had always been fascinated by the complexity of the universe. However, he struggled with finding meaning and purpose in his life. After experiencing a psychedelic trip, he felt a profound spiritual connection with the universe and finally found the answers he had been searching for. Today, Ian has a renewed sense of purpose and passion for life.

Opening the Mind

Maggie had always been curious about spirituality but struggled with finding a connection. After experiencing a psychedelic trip, she felt a sense of oneness with the universe and had a newfound understanding of the interconnectedness of all things. She describes the experience as opening her mind to new possibilities and leading her down a path of self-discovery and spiritual growth.

CHAPTER 3: PERSONAL STORIES OF HEALING

Subchapter 3.1: Overcoming Addiction

Addiction is a difficult thing to overcome, and those who have struggled with it will understand how easy it can be to relapse. However, many individuals have found success in using psychedelics to help them beat their addiction. One personal story of using psychedelics to overcome addiction is that of Jane, who was addicted to alcohol for over a decade. After several unsuccessful attempts to quit, Jane decided to try using LSD in a therapeutic setting. With a guide present, Jane experienced a profound psychedelic experience that helped her confront the underlying issues that were contributing to her addiction. Similarly, John had been struggling with opioid addiction for years. He had tried many traditional forms of treatment, such as rehab and medication-assisted therapy, but nothing seemed to work for him. Finally, John decided to try using ayahuasca, a plant-based psychedelic, to help him recover. During his ayahuasca ceremony, John experienced a sense of connection to something greater than himself, which helped him find the motivation to overcome his addiction. While these stories are anecdotal, there is promising research being conducted on the use of psychedelics in addiction treatment. Studies have shown that using psychedelics in a therapeutic setting can help individuals overcome addiction by providing them with a new perspective on their behavior and underlying issues. It is important to note that using psychedelics in this way should always be done in a controlled and safe environment with the guidance of a licensed professional. Psychedelics can be a powerful tool in addiction recovery, but they need to be used responsibly and with caution. Overall, the use of psychedelics in addiction treatment offers hope for those struggling with addiction. These substances have the potential to help individuals confront their underlying issues and gain a new perspective on their behavior, ultimately leading to a successful recovery.

CHAPTER 3: PERSONAL STORIES OF HEALING

Subchapter 3.2: Coping with Mental Illness

Mental illness is a serious issue that affects millions of people worldwide. The stigma surrounding mental health often prevents individuals from seeking the help they need. Traditional treatments, such as therapy and medication, can be effective but may not work for everyone. For some individuals, psychedelic-assisted therapy has been a transformative experience in coping with mental illness. Studies have shown that psychedelic substances, when used in a controlled setting with the guidance of a licensed therapist, can lead to significant improvements in symptoms related to depression, anxiety, PTSD, and addiction. One individual who experienced this benefit firsthand is Sarah. Sarah had been struggling with anxiety and depression since her early twenties. She had tried therapy and various medications, but nothing seemed to alleviate her symptoms. It wasn't until she heard about psychedelic-assisted therapy that she found hope. Sarah underwent a series of psychedelic therapy sessions with the guidance of a trained therapist. She described the experience as life-changing, stating that it allowed her to confront and process past traumas that had been the root cause of her mental illness. By facing these issues head-on, she was able to develop a deeper understanding of herself and gradually overcome her symptoms. Sarah's story is just one of many examples of the potential benefits of psychedelic-assisted therapy for mental illness. Of course, it's worth noting that not everyone will have the same experience, and there are risks associated with any type of drug use. However, as more research is conducted, it's becoming increasingly clear that psychedelic substances have tremendous potential as a tool for healing. In the next chapter, we'll explore the therapeutic setting in more detail, including how a licensed therapist can help guide individuals through a psychedelic experience and how follow-up care is crucial for long-term success.

CHAPTER 3: PERSONAL STORIES OF HEALING

Subchapter 3.3: Finding Spiritual Connection

Psychedelics have been known to induce spiritual experiences in users, allowing them to explore their consciousness and connect with a higher power. It has been reported that experiencing a spiritual connection can lead to feelings of peace, love, and connectedness that can have long-lasting positive effects on mental health. In several studies, participants reported that their psychedelic experience allowed them to access a sense of spirituality and connectedness that they had never felt before. Many described the experience as deeply meaningful and life-changing. One participant shared, "During my psilocybin experience, I felt a connection to something greater than myself. It was like I was part of something much bigger and more profound than anything I had ever experienced before. This connection has stayed with me, and I feel more spiritually grounded and at peace with the world." However, it's important to note that not everyone who uses psychedelics will have a spiritual experience, and that spirituality is a personal and subjective experience. It's also crucial to approach spirituality in a respectful and open-minded manner. For those who are interested in exploring spirituality through psychedelics, it's recommended to do so in a safe and controlled environment with a trained guide or therapist. A supportive and non-judgmental setting can help facilitate a positive and meaningful experience. Overall, finding a spiritual connection can be a powerful and transformative experience, and psychedelics have the potential to facilitate this journey for some individuals. However, it's important to approach spirituality with caution and respect, and to prioritize safety and responsibility throughout the psychedelic experience.

Healing in a Therapeutic Setting

Psychedelic-assisted therapy is not a do-it-yourself approach. It involves working with a guide or trained therapist in a safe and supportive environment. This chapter will explore the importance of a therapeutic setting and the ethical considerations that come with undergoing psychedelic therapy.

WORKING WITH A GUIDE

Psychedelic therapy involves working with a guide who can provide support and guidance throughout the experience. The guide helps create a safe and supportive environment that allows the participant to explore their inner thoughts and feelings.

The guide is responsible for preparing the participant before the experience and ensuring their safety during the session. They also help the participant integrate the experience into their everyday life. The guide's presence is crucial in ensuring that the experience is positive and constructive.

INTEGRATION AND FOLLOW-UP

Integration refers to the process of applying the insights gained during the psychedelic experience to everyday life. It involves exploring the emotions, thoughts, and behaviors that came up during the experience and finding ways to integrate them into daily life. Psychedelic therapy is not a quick fix. Integration takes time, patience, and commitment. Follow-up sessions with the guide or therapist can help the participant better understand and apply the insights gained during the experience.

ETHICAL CONSIDERATIONS

Psychedelic therapy is not without its ethical considerations. The therapist or guide has a responsibility to ensure the safety and well-being of the participant throughout the experience. They must also maintain the participant's confidentiality and privacy. Participants must give informed consent before the experience and have the right to withdraw from the session at any time. The therapist or guide must also be aware of any medical conditions or medications that may affect the experience. In addition, the therapist or guide must be aware of their own biases and not project them onto the participant. They must also refrain from any behaviors that may take advantage of the participant or cause harm. In conclusion, healing with psychedelics in a therapeutic setting involves working with a trained therapist or guide and engaging in a process of integration that takes time and commitment. Ethical considerations must also be taken into account to ensure the safety and well-being of the participant.

WORKING WITH A GUIDE

Psychedelic-assisted therapy always involves the presence of a guide or therapist who will guide the patient through the entire experience. This guide might often be a mental health professional or someone who has undergone extensive training in psychedelic therapy. The primary role of the guide is to create a supportive, comfortable, and safe environment for the patient and to ensure that the experience meets the patient's intentions and needs. Throughout the therapy session, the guide will act as a mediator, providing the patient with guidance and support to navigate the often intense and emotional experience. The guide usually sits with the patient during the psychedelic session, providing a presence of safety and support. Many patients who have undergone psychedelic-assisted therapy often describe the guide as an integral part of the experience, providing much-needed guidance and support. The guide may also work with the patient before the psychedelic session to prepare them for the experience. This preparation may involve psychotherapy sessions to discuss the patient's intentions, fears, and expectations. The guide may also advise the patient on how to manage their expectations and make important changes in their life. The guide may also help the patient integrate the experience into their daily life after the psychedelic session. The guide offers support, helps the patient process the experience and provides guidance on how to apply the insights and lessons they have gained from the experience in their daily life. Working with a guide is an essential aspect of the psychedelic-assisted therapy process. The presence of an experienced guide can create a supportive and safe environment for the patient, which can enhance the healing potential of the experience. With the right guide, patients can undergo psychedelic therapy safely and with a greater chance of achieving their therapeutic goals. It is important to note that psychedelics are potent substances, and their use must be approached with caution and respect. Patients must undergo psychedelic-assisted therapy only under the supervision of an experienced guide in a safe and supportive environment.

CHAPTER 4: HEALING IN A THERAPEUTIC SETTING

Subchapter 4.2: Integration and Follow-Up

Psychedelic-assisted therapy has shown immense promise in treating addiction, depression, anxiety, and other mental health conditions. However, the journey to healing is not complete once the psychedelic experience is over. Integration and follow-up care are critical aspects of the healing process. Integration involves taking the insights and revelations gained during the psychedelic experience and incorporating them into daily life. It can be challenging to navigate this process on your own, which is why integration therapy is often a critical component of psychedelic-assisted therapy. Integration therapy involves meeting with a therapist to discuss the psychedelic experience and how it can be integrated into daily life. The therapist can help identify patterns and behaviors that may be obstructing the healing process and provide guidance on how to make positive changes. Follow-up care is also essential for individuals who have undergone psychedelic therapy. Follow-up care involves regular check-ins with the therapist to ensure that progress is being made and to address any new issues that may arise. It can also involve revisiting the psychedelic experience to deepen healing or explore new insights. It is essential to prioritize integration and follow-up care, as they can have a significant impact on the long-term success of psychedelic-assisted therapy. By receiving ongoing support, individuals can ensure that they are making the most of their psychedelic experience and continuing to benefit from its insights and healing potential. In conclusion, integration and follow-up care are critical components of the healing process with psychedelics. They can help individuals translate insights gained during the psychedelic experience into meaningful changes in their daily lives. Ongoing support from a therapist can ensure that progress is being made and new challenges are addressed, leading to long-term healing and recovery.

CHAPTER 4: HEALING IN A THERAPEUTIC SETTING

Subchapter 4.3: Ethical Considerations

As the use of psychedelics in therapeutic settings becomes more common, it is important to consider the ethical implications of this type of treatment. While there are many potential benefits to using psychedelics for healing and recovery, there are also risks and potential harms that must be taken into account. One of the primary ethical considerations when using psychedelics in therapy is the issue of informed consent. It is essential that patients fully understand the risks and benefits of psychedelic-assisted therapy before they participate in it. This means providing patients with detailed information about the potential risks of using psychedelics, as well as the potential benefits. Patients should also be informed about the legal status of psychedelics and the potential consequences of using them outside of a therapeutic setting. Another important ethical consideration is the need to ensure that patients are not exploited or taken advantage of in any way. This means that therapists must have the best interests of the patient at heart and must not use psychedelic-assisted therapy for personal gain or profit. Therapists must also be trained and experienced in working with psychedelics and must be able to provide a safe and supportive environment for their patients. Confidentiality is another important ethical consideration when it comes to psychedelic-assisted therapy. Patients must be assured that their personal information will be kept confidential and that their privacy will be respected at all times. This means that therapists must take care to keep their patients' information confidential, while also taking steps to protect their patients' safety and well-being. Finally, it is important to consider the societal implications of using psychedelics in therapy. While psychedelics have the potential to be a powerful tool for healing and recovery, there is also the risk that their use could be stigmatized or misunderstood by the wider community. It is important for therapists and patients alike to be aware of the potential risks and benefits of using psychedelics in therapy and to work to reduce stigma and increase understanding of this type of treatment. In conclusion, there are many important ethical considerations to take into account when using psychedelics in therapeutic settings. By ensuring that patients are fully informed and protected, that therapists are experienced and responsible, and that confidentiality and societal implications are carefully considered, we can help to ensure that psychedelic-assisted therapy is used in a safe, responsible, and effective way.

Chapter 5: Moving Forward

With the increasing amount of research on the benefits of psychedelics for mental health treatment, it's essential to advocate for necessary changes. The potential of psychedelic-assisted therapy is immense, and it's essential to keep pushing for more research, more legalization, and more acceptance. In this chapter, we'll discuss how to move forward with psychedelic-assisted therapy.

SUBCHAPTER 5.1: ADVOCATING FOR CHANGE

One way to advocate for change is by educating people about the benefits of psychedelic-assisted therapy. When people understand how these substances can help people overcome addiction, PTSD, depression, and anxiety, they may be more likely to support its legalization. Starting conversations about the topic and sharing personal stories can help spread awareness. Another way to advocate for change is by contacting local politicians and expressing support for psychedelic-assisted therapy. Find out who your elected officials are and write letters or emails explaining why this type of treatment is essential. The more support they receive from their constituents, the more likely they are to take action.

Subheading 5.1.1: The Power of Grassroots Movements

Grassroots movements can be a powerful tool for advocacy. It's possible to organize rallies, protests, and events to draw attention to the cause. Social media can also be used to spread awareness and help people connect with one another. By coming together, we can create a powerful voice for change.

SUBCHAPTER 5.2: FUTURE OF PSYCHEDELIC-ASSISTED THERAPY

The future of psychedelic-assisted therapy is hopeful. As more research is conducted, we'll learn more about how psychedelic substances can be used to treat a variety of mental health issues. With more openness to the idea of these substances and more advocates pushing for legalization, it's possible that psychedelic-assisted therapy will become more widely available in therapeutic settings.

Subheading 5.2.1: Establishing Guidelines and Standards

As psychedelic-assisted therapy becomes more widespread, it's necessary to establish guidelines and standards for its use. Ethical considerations, such as how to ensure patient safety and how to prevent abuse of psychedelic substances, must be addressed. It's crucial to work with trained professionals who follow established procedures for administering these substances to achieve the best outcomes.

SUBCHAPTER 5.3: CONCLUSION AND FINAL THOUGHTS

Overall, psychedelic-assisted therapy offers hope for those who have struggled with mental health issues. It's essential to continue advocating for change and promoting awareness of the potential benefits of this type of therapy. With the right guidance and the right approach, psychedelic substances can be a powerful tool for healing and recovery. Let's keep pushing forward and breaking the stigma surrounding this life-changing therapy.

ADVOCATING FOR CHANGE

The stigma surrounding psychedelic drugs has been deeply ingrained in our society for decades. However, as more and more research is conducted on the therapeutic potential of these drugs, it is becoming increasingly clear that they could be a game-changer in the field of mental health treatment. One of the most important ways to break the stigma is to educate the public. Many people still associate psychedelics with the counterculture of the 1960s and view them as dangerous and illegal drugs. Advocates for the therapeutic use of psychedelics need to work to change this perception by sharing accurate information and data. One way to do this is to support and fund further research into the therapeutic benefits of psychedelics. The more evidence we have to support their use in treating mental health conditions, the more likely it is that the medical community and the general public will take notice. Another important step is to try to change laws and regulations that currently prevent people from accessing these potentially life-saving treatments. While some progress has been made in recent years, there is still a long way to go. Advocates could lobby their elected officials, write letters to local and national news outlets, and start grassroots campaigns to raise awareness. Finally, it is important to support organizations that are working to change perceptions and regulations surrounding psychedelics. These organizations can provide valuable resources and information to those who are interested in learning more about psychedelics and their potential as a therapeutic tool. As more and more people share their own personal stories of healing and recovery with psychedelics, the stigma surrounding these drugs will continue to crumble. Advocating for change is a vital part of this process, and it is a responsibility that should not be taken lightly. By working together, we can help to create a world where psychedelic-assisted therapy is seen as a legitimate and effective treatment option for those who need it most.

SUBCHAPTER 5.2: FUTURE OF PSYCHEDELIC-ASSISTED THERAPY

The future of psychedelic-assisted therapy is bright, with ongoing research providing promising results. As more studies are conducted and more people experience the benefits of these substances, it is likely that they will become more widely accepted and available for therapeutic use. One potential area of growth is through the use of telemedicine and online therapy. With the COVID-19 pandemic forcing people to stay at home and limit in-person interactions, the use of virtual therapy sessions has become more widespread. While psychedelic-assisted therapy is still largely conducted in person, there is potential for online sessions to be an effective tool in expanding access and reaching more people. Another area of potential growth is through the development of new substances. While LSD and psilocybin have been at the forefront of psychedelic-assisted therapy, there are many other naturally occurring and synthetic substances that could be explored for therapeutic use. For example, research is currently being conducted on the use of ibogaine for addiction treatment, and ayahuasca for depression and anxiety. Finally, there is potential for the legalization and regulation of psychedelic substances. As more evidence is gathered supporting their use in therapy, it is possible that these substances could be legalized for medical use and regulated in a similar manner to other prescription drugs. This would allow for increased access and safety in therapeutic settings. In conclusion, the future of psychedelic-assisted therapy is exciting and full of potential. As more research is conducted and more people experience the benefits of these substances, it is likely that they will become more widely accepted and available for therapeutic use. The expansion of virtual therapy sessions, the exploration of new substances, and the potential for legalization and regulation all point towards a bright future for psychedelic-assisted therapy.

www.ingramcontent.com/pod-product-compliance
Lightning Source LLC
Chambersburg PA
CBHW061526250726
48657CB00005B/2100